HERBALISM

----- ✤✤✤✤ -----

*Live a long healthy life with natural
herbs for healing and dieting purposes*

Kirsten Yang

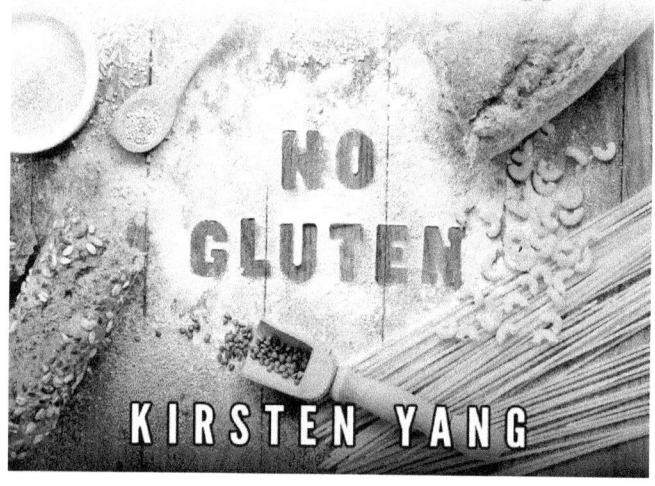

Do you have celiac disease or gluten sensitivity?
This book will show you just how tasty a gluten-free diet can be.

CLICK HERE AND GET YOUR COPY NOW

https://goo.gl/kf1fJo

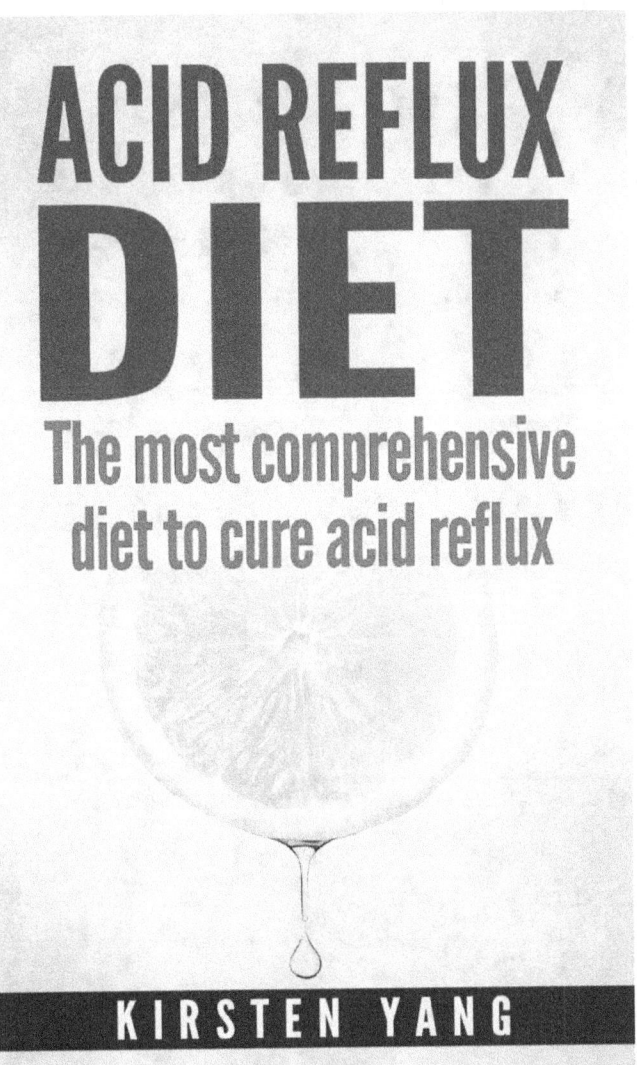

Do you wanna stop the acid reflux with the ultimate cookbook and feel free to talk with people!?

CLICK HERE AND GET YOUR COPY NOW

https://goo.gl/GFyrH1

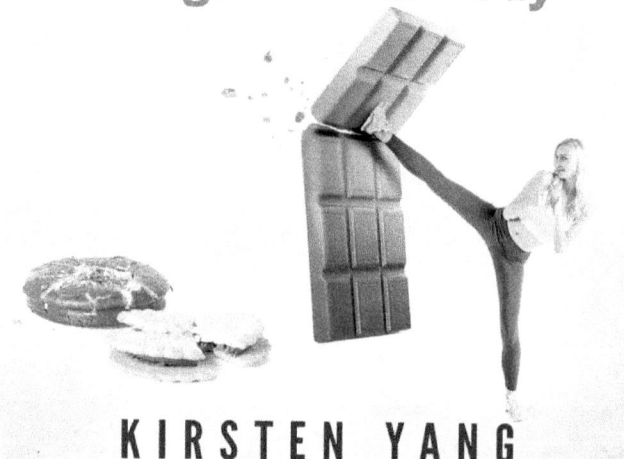

liable for any hardship or damages that may befall them after undertaking information described herein.

Additionally, the information in the following pages is intended only for informational purposes and should thus be thought of as universal. As befitting its nature, it is presented without assurance regarding its prolonged validity or interim quality. Trademarks that are mentioned are done without written consent and can in no way be considered an endorsement from the trademark holder.

TABLE OF CONTENT

INTRODUCTION

It's important to remember that everything that exists in modern medicine is derived from things we've found correctly in nature.

Herbal remedies to medical issues have been around since the time in which man first held any understanding whatsoever of the vulnerabilities of his own anatomy.

The study of herbalism has evolved in parallel, in many ways, to our overall understanding of nature. While many people in the medical profession don't take it seriously, the truth is that what has come to evolve over the course of many centuries is a robust system of alternative medicine that provides a wide range of solutions for any number of ailments.

The beauty of the study of Herbalism is that mankind has even had to do a lot of work in order to turn substances found in nature into something that's useful in medicine. Nature does a lot of the work for us through the sheer diversity of the plants that grow in different regions of the world, and the organic solutions that are held within them that have myriad medical applications.

The hard part, from the perspective of an herbalist, is simply one where to look. Although a lot of ingredients in today's medicines are artificially synthesized, very sizable portions of what goes into today's pharmaceutical solutions to literally thousands of ailments are derived from fully natural, botanical substances.

In areas of the world where they reach of modern pharmaceutical organizations has not been able to have a lot of influence, herbalism is still one of the predominant forms of medicine in practice. The study of herbalism in many ways requires just as much discipline is the study of modern medicinal techniques. Since the range of floral offerings is great, patients leave themselves open to the possibility that a botanical solution can have negative effects on their condition just as easily as it can have positive effects.

The benefits of herbalism are primarily twofold. First, if you are properly diagnosed and the herbal solution is recommended for your treatment, the likelihood of side effects causing inconveniences in your life is relatively low compared to other types of medicine.

If you don't believe that, just take a look at any commercial, for a medical pill that you see on television, and the first thing you'll notice is that half the commercial is dedicated to listing out all the side effects that can possibly happen to you.

When you think about it, that sounds more like a solution to a problem that just creates more problems.

The second benefit to herbalism is the cost. Natural remedies have been around for thousands of years longer than modern pharmaceutical companies have, in many forms of this folk medicine have been passed down as family remedies for ailments, all of which can be pieced together from things you can find in nature for extremely little cost.

This is one of the biggest reasons why it's so popular in areas of the world that have never heard of things like "universal health care." It works well enough for them, and should never be ignored as a potential solution to problems in our Western civilization.

CHAPTER 1:

WHAT IS HERBALISM?

Herbalism is a traditional medical practice based on the use of plants and their extracts.

Herbalism is also referred to as physiotherapy, botanical medicine, herbal medicine, medical herbalism, herbology, and medicinal botany. In addition to plants, herbalism occasionally includes bee products, shells, certain animal parts, and even fungi.

Herbalism is the treatment of various ailments through natural sources found in the various plant life available. Although it may sound a bit primitive, it forms the basis of modern pharmaceutical medicine in many ways.

Often considered and derided as a form of folk medicine, herbalism is something you, me and everyone generally practices whether we realize it or not. It is simply the use of certain plants to relieve a particular ailment.

When you take aspirin for a headache, you are essentially practicing herbalism in a sense. Why? Aspirin comes from the inner bark of the Willow tree. Obviously, it does not come in the form of a tablet, but there is no denying the relief you obtain from taking it is from the plant derivative of that bark.

CHAPTER 1: WHAT IS HERBALISM?

While it is true that most remedies come from natural sources, the modern definition of herbalism is much more restrictive than what we have suggested to this point.

It is more about the direct rendering of herbs to a medicinal form where an industrial manufacturer of pills is not involved. This form of herbalism has a long history. From 3000 BC, we have records of Sumerians using thyme to treat ailments. The first herbalism book is believed to be one found in China and dating from 2700 BC. This book is of great interest and importance. Why? It listed over 365 herbs and their medicinal properties. One was Ma Huang, which you probably know better today as Ephedrine.

The popularity of herbalism cannot be understated. From the Greeks to the Romans to the Chinese's and beyond, herbalism formed the basis of medicine through much of the world.

It was only in the 17th century that it began to lose its dominant position as a modern medicine slowly started to create new forms of treatment and distractions of plant medicinal properties into hybrid medications.

Does this mean herbalism is dead or should be avoided as a form of medicinal treatment these days? Of course not.

Pharmaceutical companies spend vast amounts of money sending people into the rain forests for a reason. They are looking for that next great drug that will revolutionize the world.

On a more practical level, herbalism has a definite place in your daily life. Herbal medicines tend to be better for you than modern alternatives because they do not contain the additives you find with pharmaceuticals.

This makes them better for you, but also easier to take as they are often mixed with teas and so on.

Is herbalism for you? Only you can answer that. Just understand that it herbalism is not some extreme fad or something weird. It formed the basis of medicine in our world for such a long period of time that one must wonder how different the world would look today had it not been discovered.

CHAPTER 2:

WHAT HERBAL HEALTH IS ALL ABOUT?

To most people herbs are thought of in terms of enhancing flavor in cooking. People also think of herbs is a reference to natural medicine and oriental medicine.

A very common use of the term herbal is in relation to herbal teas. Actually, a herb can be any plant. Herbal health is all about using specific plants (herbs) that have specific known compounds that are used in natural health and as a medicine.

While herbal health may be thought of as using herbs like some form of medicine, herbs are also whole foods that support holistic health. When I think of herb for health I feel it is the idea of using edible plants that have powerful nutritional healing and holistic health benefits to balance the body.

Often it seems herbs are mystified as being exotic potions or drug-like compounds that only very specific practitioners or healers know how to use.

While there is some truth to this, especially with formulas and combinations of herbs, there is are also a whole range of herbs used for herbal health that is easily understood.

HERBAL HEALTH IS A MODALITY FOR CREATING AND SUPPORTING OPTIMAL HEALTH.

In China and in many cultures all over the world herbal remedies have successfully been used to promote health since the dawn of man. Herbal health has been around forever and has been widely accepted by past and present societies all over the world. Yet there does continue to be a mistrust and a lot of misinformation about herbal health that persists in the U.S. culture.

Ignorance is partly to blame but there is also a concerted effort on the part of the American medical industry and the pharmaceutical industry to limit and repress the knowledge and use of herbal health therapies and medicinal herbs.

Natural medicine remedies, cures, and therapies are often very inexpensive and because they do not offer the massive profits of the drug and medical industry infrastructure they are repressed.

The government plays into this as well through the lobby influence of these industries. There have been ongoing efforts by these industries in collusion with the FDA and other governmental agencies to suppress and even ban the use of herbs for health and for the treatment of illness and disease.

Recently there have even been attempts to criminalize natural medicine practitioners and their use of herbal therapies.

The reality of herbal health is that herbs have been used for centuries to improve and maintain health and to cure illness and disease. As we look at the U.S. western medicine, health care system today, we see that the U.S. population has evolved into one of the unhealthiest on this planet, while at the same time being the wealthiest and most well fed.

The western conventional health system is heavily based on the use of pharmaceutical drugs to chase symptoms with no effective understanding our program for preventative health. People wait till they are ill, then they are put on drugs to maintain their illness and often told to take the drugs for the rest of their lives. No actual healing or cure ever takes place.

Herbal health is based on a holistic health model that uses natural medicine and nutrition as a preventative process to avoid illness and disease.

If people do get sick then the herbal health model uses herbs for natural medicine and nutrition to heal by rebalancing the body.

Healing and curing can mean the same thing or can be two different perceptions. If you are healed of an illness or imbalance then you no longer have the illness or imbalance this is the same as saying you are cured.

There are some limited occasions where you are cured with medicine or a process without going through a healing process. Like the use of an antidote, surgery or a serum that automatically cures your specific illness. Actually, outright automatic cures are rare, most illness and disease is about healing.

Illness and disease are caused or allowed to develop from imbalances in the body's systems. The use of herbs or natural health processes to create and maintain vibrant health and prevent illness and disease has actually proven to be far more effective over time than the conventional western medical model.

As long as massive profit is available for health care, illness, and disease, then people will be misinformed and prevented from using the herbal health model.

Herbs are an inexpensive form of effective medicine, for maintaining optimal health and for illness and disease prevention. Whole herbal superfoods are herbs that have been concentrated and prepared for consumption as a supplement to your normal everyday diet.

Amazon rainforest raw herbal supplements are eaten by people all over the world and the same herbs gathered and eaten in their natural wild state have been used to support the health of indigenous people in the Amazon for thousands of years.

Take a closer look at herbal superfood supplements, herbal medicines and whole foods as medicine.

If you want to be healthy naturally and prevent illness and disease before it can happen to you, then herbal health is worth investigating.

CHAPTER 3:

IDENTIFYING THE DIFFERENT FORMS OF HERBAL MEDICINE

Although there are a lot of positive things to be said when it comes to herbal medicine, is still an undeniable fact however that what we proof we have is not yet enough to make taking herbal medicine completely safe.

Hence, when you're about to try out herbal, medicine please make sure to check with your doctor first if what you're doing wouldn't be harmful to your body. Secondly, it's better to be able to identify the different forms of herbal medicine so you'd know if what you're taking is the real thing or not.

1. Essence: This is also one of the most popular forms that herbal medicine takes. Herbs with essential oils are processed through cold pressing or steam distillation.

   This form of herbal medicine is popular because a lot of people prefer to enjoy massages with the use of essential oils because it supposedly helps them relax more easily.

2. Pills and Capsules: People who violently resist the idea of taking herbal medicine in its raw form may find other products of herbal medicine in the form of pills and capsules.

    Herbal medicine is ground into powder to take this particular form. Usually, with this form of herbal medicine, the medicinal purpose is general and not meant to be a specific cure. Ampalaya capsules, for example, are taken simply to help improve your diabetes.

3. Infusions: This process involves the delicate parts of a plant like its leaves, seeds, and fruits. The process simply takes several minutes to finish.

4. Poultice: There are some situations that require patients to take herbal medicine in the form of a poultice. In this case, the herbs are macerated or chopped into tiny pieces and are then directly applied to the skin. After this, a hot, moist bandage is used to cover the area.

5. Raw: It's like going back to the primitive past when you're required to take this particular form of herbal medicine. Not only is the process somewhat undesirable, the taste it leaves nothing to be desired as well. Many health care professionals, however, advise people to step these raw herbs into tea because it's said to release its healing powers effectively.

6. Tinctures: Herbal medicine in liquid form.

7. Decoctions: This process involves the extraction of certain parts of a plant like the berries, roots, and herb-bark. This process usually takes 45 minutes to an hour and a half.

THE BENEFITS OF HERBAL MEDICINES AND TREATMENT

In today's fast moving world when everyone is chasing the money and have no time for the health, the diseases are inevitable. Nowadays, we hear about the name of the diseases which were not even existed 5 to 10 years before.

These new diseases created a number of new treatments and medicines, and almost all of these treatments are having their side effects. That is the reason now people are looking for a natural, herbal way of curing the disease.

People are looking for natural remedies instead of homeopathic, allopathic or any surgical curing process. These herbal medicines or treatments are not a new thing, but they are in existence for thousands of years. The main advantages of these medicines are that they are not having any kind of side effects at all unlike those of allopathic medicines.

Unlike those fast healing medicines available in the market, herbal drugs may take some time to cure the disease, but it will not leave any kind of side effects. According to some market research companies, the market of herbal remedies is increasing by 25-30% a year, which is one of the fastest-growing alternative health industry.

ADVANTAGES OF HERBAL MEDICINES

1. PRICE

Herbal medicines are a way cheaper as compared to their allopathic or homeopathic counterpart. Also, it is very safe to take the herbal medicines without the prescription of any Doctor, unlike the other medicines.

CHAPTER 3: IDENTIFYING THE DIFFERENT FORMS OF HERBAL MEDICINE

Also the main problem with regular allopathic or homeopathic medicines is that if you are taking this kind of medicines for a particular problem, for example, if you are taking any medicine for back pain, and now you are suffering from fever then you have to take a good precaution so that both of these medicines cannot be in conflict.

Herbal medicines do not follow under the category of the drug instead they fall under the category of food. Herbal medicines can also be termed as a food supplement thus not subjected to the same kind of scientific prescription and inspection.

2. EFFECTIVENESS

The main reason behind that the people are looking for these herbs that they are either this is dissatisfied with their regular kind of medicines/remedies, or they are suffering from some kind of side effect at these remedies.

However, the main problem with the herbal medicines is that the fewer numbers of companies are interested in the manufacturing herbal medicines. Thus, it is sometimes difficult to find out the herbal medicine of a reputed company.

However, this trend is changing rapidly and a lot of reputed companies are stepping into the manufacturing of herbal medicines.

Being sick isn't cheap nowadays. Most drug companies know that people will pay anything just to avail the drugs needed to alleviate from illness. Their tag prices that are off the roof and consumer have no choice but to pay.

That's why alternative medicine has come up ways to combat this injustice by releasing herbal supplements that are cheap, convenient, effective, and available to all.

REASONS WHY YOU SHOULD OPT FOR HERBAL SUPPLEMENTS BEFORE IT'S TOO LATE

1. HERBAL MEDICINE HAVE BEEN TESTED AND PROVEN THROUGHOUT TIME

Little did we know that herbal medicine has been around ever since man can record it? There are numerous accounts in different parts of the world that herbal medicine has been constantly used for its effectiveness and convenience. Cultures governing Asia all the way to Europe have various techniques and ways of preparing herbal medicines that have saved their civilization throughout the ages. This strongly proves the effectiveness of herbal medicines.

2. NO SIDE EFFECTS

Because herbal medicines are naturally made, safe and effective, there are no side effects. For the past decade, there have been no reported fatal side effects with regards to the use of herbal supplements. It is 100% for all ages, from kids, teens, adults and the elderly.

Now, everyone can live a happy, normal and productive life thanks to herbal medicines.

3. NO WORRIES ABOUT OVERDOSAGE

You don't have to worry about overdosing anymore. Since herbal medicines are all-natural and safe, even if you took more than the normal dosage, your body will just flush out the excess supplements taken via urine.

This won't even harm your filtering organ like liver, kidneys and such. You don't worry about taking it with a full stomach or not either. It isn't harmful to the stomach's wall and inner lining and it doesn't react much with the acid inside.

4. HERBAL SUPPLEMENTS ARE INSANELY CHEAPER

Another vital way in order to live a healthy life is to take in supplements. Commercially prepared supplements nowadays are too costly and practical-wise, I'd rather buy milk and eggs for my family rather than buying supplements. This is not true for herbal supplements. They are much cheaper, even compared to the prices a carton of milk and a tray of eggs.

They are so affordable that everyone in the family can take one every day to sustain the body at its optimal level of functioning.

In this way, you'll be protecting your family from illnesses and keeping you from paying insanely high hospital bills, doctor's consultation fees, and overpriced medications. Consider this the next time you buy groceries.

You have to worry about its credibility either. These herbal supplements are regulated by the FDA. They wouldn't be sold in the market publicly if it hasn't gone through the watchful eyes of the FDA. There certain FDA logos attached to the bottle or brand, if you want to check it out.

5. STUDIES PROVIDES EVIDENCE ON THE EFFICACY OF HERBAL SUPPLEMENTS

There are thousands of pages on the Internet making claims about the effectiveness of herbal supplements. Various companies, universities, and other health institutions had started the using herbal supplements are 100% safe and effective, not to mention cheap.

Try to consider choosing herbal supplements rather than sticking to commercially prepared medications that can cause harmful side effects.

It is much safer to invest in something safer rather than taking risks that may cause much harm than good. All natural remedies are taking the country by storm and it's about time that you jump in as well. Start living, health right now by having a proper balanced diet, ample amount of exercise, enough rest and sleep and taking herbal supplements to boost your immunity, protecting you from sickness and keeping your body at its optimum level of functioning.

CHAPTER 4:

PRECAUTIONS AND TIPS BEFORE USING HERBAL SUPPLEMENTS

The list of herbal remedies goes ceaselessly. Herbal remedies aren't new; plants have been used for medicinal purposes for thousands of years. Though, herbal supplements have not been subjected to the same scientific analysis and aren't as sternly regulated as medications.

For example, herbal supplement manufacturers don't have to get authorization from the Food and Drug Administration previous to putting their goods on the market.

PRECAUTIONS

Up till now several herbal supplements- together with products labeled as "natural" - have drug-like effects that can be hazardous. So it's important to investigate prospective benefits and side effects of herbal supplements before you purchase.

And be confident to talk with your doctor before trying herbal supplements. In fact, in some high-risk situations, your doctor will likely suggest that you avoid herbal supplements overall.

CHAPTER 4: PRECAUTIONS AND TIPS BEFORE USING HERBAL SUPPLEMENTS

You may be introducing yourself at risk by using herbal supplements if:

- You're taking prescription: Some herbs can grounds serious side effects when diverse with prescription and OTC drugs such as aspirin, blood pressure or blood thinner medications. Talk to your doctor about feasible exchanges.

- You're pregnant: Medications that may be secure for you as a grown person may be dangerous to your fetus. As a common rule, don't take any medications prescription, OTC or herbal when you're breastfeeding except your doctor approves.

- You're having an operation: Many herbal can influence the triumph of surgery. Some may decrease the efficiency of anesthetics or cause hazardous complications, such as high blood pressure or bleeding.

  Tell your doctor regarding any herbs you're taking or allowing for taking as soon as you know you need surgery.

- You're younger than 18 or bigger than 65- Older adults may metabolize medications in a different way. And few herbal supplements have been tested on children or have recognized safe doses for kids.

SAFETY TIPS FOR USING HERBAL SUPPLEMENTS

- Trail supplement information: Don't exceed suggested dosages or take the herb for longer than suggested.

- Keep trail of what you take: Take only one supplement at a time to settle on if it's effectual. Compose a note of what you get and how much for how long; and how it affects you.

- Avoid products with a ruined past: A number of herbal weight-loss pills have been found to have solemn side effects or to contain prescription drugs or contaminants. For this reason, they're almost certainly best avoided.

- Test alerts and advisories- The FDA and NCCAM continue lists of supplements that are under authoritarian review or that have been reported to cause poor effects. Check their Websites occasionally for updates.

CHAPTER 5:

WHY CHOOSE HERBAL VITAMINS?

Including herbal vitamins as part of your health and wellness regimen is a powerful preventative measure against disease and aging. As we age, we begin to look for ways to ensure the best of health as we grow older.

The idea is to be energetic and self-reliant as we transition into our golden years before we need to rely on dangerous drugs to control age-related illnesses and conditions.

Modern pharmaceuticals are rarely used for preventative measures in the same way as herbal vitamins. In other words, they are prescribed only for a specific medical condition has been diagnosed.

Sure, your doctor might prescribe blood pressure lowering medication to prevent stroke, but wouldn't it be better to give your body a chance to prevent high blood pressure in the first place? Heart medication is given to those who are already at risk for heart attack. How about taking steps to prevent the risk in the first place?

And with the recent concerns over the safety and side-effects of modern pharmaceutical drugs, many people are looking for herbal vitamins as a source for health, wellness, and longevity.

No one can guarantee that you won't develop high blood pressure or cancer or some other life-threatening condition, but herbal vitamins can give your body the best chance at avoiding these conditions. The benefits of herbal dietary supplements are well-documented.

They have a very low occurrence of side-effects, they are gentler on the body, and have been used by ancient civilizations for generations. Their popularity continues to grow today.

I should also point out that the term herbal vitamins do not refer only to vitamins (such as vitamin A, B, C, etc.), but to all compounds that make up herbal remedies. Herbs contain far more ingredients than isolated vitamins, which is one of the reasons they are so powerful.

Scientists have been delving into herbal vitamins for years, attempting to isolate the specific chemicals that have these positive effects on our health and well-being.

They are finding that while certain chemicals do seem to have beneficial effects, herbal whole food supplements that contain all of the components of the herbs from which they originate seems to be the most effective in many cases.

And now that human DNA has been decoded, genetic researchers are also beginning to embrace herbal vitamins, and we are seeing the companies now to offer complete herbal dietary supplements that are custom tailored to an individual's unique DNA.

This is a revolutionary breakthrough in nutritional research and a huge step forward in natural preventative care.

Including herbal supplements as part of your overall health and wellness regimen is a smart move.

While no one can guarantee, exactly how you will age, or what conditions you will get over time, herbal vitamins will help ensure that your body has best opportunities to maintain good health. Modern pharmaceuticals have their uses, but they are not good long-term solutions and are not intended for preventative care.

Remember, everyone's needs are different, so be sure to choose herbal vitamins that match your body's needs. Base your choices on your own personal history or the history of family members.

If you want the most targeted nutrition possible, with the least amount of guesswork, get your DNA tested and have a custom formula created just for you.

HERBAL VITAMINS FOR A HEALTHIER YOU

Herbal supplements and vitamin supplements are often interchanged. Most herbs contain some vitamins. Vitamins are usually either synthetic or derived from animals, herbs or fruit. From this close association, the concept of herbal vitamins emerged.

THE NEED FOR VITAMINS

Since our bodies cannot manufacture or synthesize most of the identified vitamins, we must get vitamins from outside sources. When we use the phrase "herbal vitamins", we are typically referring to vitamins that have been derived from herbs. Like any other vitamins, herbal vitamins are taken as either a dietary component or a dietary supplement.

WHAT DO HERBAL VITAMINS?

Vitamins, whether derived from herbs or from another source, are essential to the proper functioning of the human body. Herbal vitamins can provide support to the human body in the forms of healthy growth, vitality and overall health.

However, don't fall for the belief that herbal vitamins can be a replacement for healthy food.

In fact, most experts now believe that the body can't properly use even herbal vitamins without the other components that typically accompany these vitamins in healthy foods.

That is why it is usually recommended that you take your herbal vitamins with a meal, one that is preferably healthy.

One of the main functions that these herbal vitamins are intended to assist in is the regulation of metabolism. They help in transforming fat and carbohydrates into a form that the cells can use. Also, vitamins are believed to aid in the proper formation of bones and tissue.

HERBS RICH IN BETA-CAROTENE

Perhaps one of the best examples of herbal vitamins is beta-carotene, which the body converts to vitamin A. The human body uses vitamin A in order to aid the growth and repair of body tissues. Many herbs contain beta carotene.

The herb is known as agrimony, or what many people refer to as "plant healing to eyes", is a particularly good herbal source of beta-carotene. Herbal skin care treatments usually have beta-carotene in hopes of maintaining smooth, soft, disease-free skin. Vitamin A converted from herbal vitamins can be used by the body to counteract night blindness and weak eyesight.

Another popular herbal vitamin is Vitalerbs. It can be found in many health food stores and nutrition centers. It is composed of herbs such as alfalfa, dandelion, kelp and purple duce.

Because the vitamins remain intact with their herbal sources, the body is more able to absorb and put the vitamins contained in it to use. It contains many vitamins in their natural form such as ascorbic acid, biotin, calcium, choline, and pantothenic acid, iodine and iron.

CHAPTER 6:

HERBAL NUTRITION SUPPLEMENTS

Herbal nutrition supplements are everywhere these days. So should you be taking them? To help you decide for yourself, here are the who's, what's, when's, where and whys on herbal nutrition.

1. HERBAL NUTRITION SUPPLEMENTS: WHAT ARE THEY?

The National Library of Medicine gives this definition: "Herbal supplements are a type of dietary supplement... that contains herbs, either singly or in mixtures".

Herbal nutrition supplements come in a variety of different forms, however, and some are better and safer than others.

2. QUALITY HERBAL SUPPLEMENTS: WHY TAKE THEM?

There is a good chance that quality herbal supplements may be a healthy choice for you. Herbal nutrition supplements are excellent for people who are unable to meet their nutritional requirements because of food allergies, medical conditions, or busy schedules that don't leave enough time to control and monitor nutrient intake.

3. QUALITY NATURAL SUPPLEMENTS: WHO SHOULD TAKE THEM?

Herbal nutrition supplements can be very beneficial for a wide range of people who need to fill in the nutritional gaps left by an incomplete diet.

However, there are also people who should not take herbal nutrition supplements. Check with your doctor first if you have:

- High blood pressure

- Thyroid problems

- Parkinson's disease

- An enlarged prostate gland

- Blood clotting problems

- Diabetes

- Heart disease

- Epilepsy

- Glaucoma

- History of stroke

- Liver problems Or, if you are pregnant or nursing

4. HERBAL NUTRITION SUPPLEMENTS: WHEN SHOULD YOU TAKE THEM?

Herbal nutrition supplements can serve as a great complement to your diet or as an addition to conventional medicine. It's important to note, however, that in some cases, combining herbal nutrition supplements with other medicine can be lethal.

If you're currently taking any doctor prescribed or over-the-counter medicine, be sure to consult your doctor before taking any herbal nutrition supplements.

5. QUALITY HERBAL SUPPLEMENTS: WHERE DO YOU FIND THEM?

Herbal nutrition supplements are not all created equal. Be extremely cautioned. Your best bet is to stick to well-known products with wide usage and a popular history.

Herbal nutrition supplements, when used by the right person, at the right time can have incredible health benefits.

WHY HERBAL DIETARY SUPPLEMENTS ARE SO POPULAR

Herbal dietary supplements are commonly used today by an increasing number of people to treat various health conditions and diseases. As the name suggests, herbal supplements are those that contain herbs or botanical ingredients.

Herbal dietary supplements are so popular because they provide a natural and healthy solution for improving one's health and quality of life.

CHAPTER 6: HERBAL NUTRITION SUPPLEMENTS

Many people are under the impression that herbal dietary supplements are new additions to the health industry. However, in reality, the use of herbs and medicine go back to prehistoric man.

1. GUIDELINES THAT SUPPLEMENTS SHOULD FOLLOW

There are certain guidelines that herbal dietary supplements have to fulfill by its manufacturers. They should be taken orally to supplement the diet by increasing one's dietary daily intake. Most herbal dietary supplements contain one or more vitamins, herbs, minerals and amino acids to maintain the body's nutritional balance.

Different supplements are available in different forms like capsule, powder, pill, gel caps, liquids and concentrate soft gels for quick and easy absorption of the supplement in the body.

2. NOT A MEAL ON ITS OWN

However, remember that herbal dietary supplements are in no way a conventional food or meal supplement that can be taken on its own.

It is to be included in your diet with your regular food, as a nutritional and beneficial supplement. With there being different types of herbal supplements, more than 5 billion people take some form of herbal supplements in their day to day life.

The most common reasons for people to take these supplements include prevention of some disease or illness, to help with weight loss, for the improvement of one's energy levels and to cure insomnia or to help one relax and sleep.

Herbal supplements are also taken to manage any symptoms that arise due to illness, injury or disease and to increase one's life longevity. Sometimes it is also used as a part or alternative to traditional medicinal treatments or even as an alternative to the more expensive treatments.

3. CONSULT YOUR DOCTOR

Some people use herbal supplements only because they are a convenient means of adding some vitamins, minerals, and herbs in their diet. Then again, there are people who take these supplements just to improve their performance in their physical, emotional and mental well-being.

So you can see that herbal dietary supplements are indeed very beneficial in improving your health and general well-being.

However, just like any other medication, it is always better to consult your physician or doctor about taking these supplements, especially if you suffer from other health ailments like diabetes and high blood pressure.

CHAPTER 7:

HERBAL REMEDIES FOR BETTER HEALTH AND HORMONE BALANCE

Conventional medicine is responsible for 255,000 deaths per year in the United States, and almost half of those are from adverse reactions to prescription drugs.

Just because a pharmaceutical drug has been studied in a laboratory, regulated by the FDA and prescribed by a doctor, it does not necessarily mean that it is safe - especially mixing with other Rx drugs.

Of course, modern medicine can be safe, effective and has certainly saved millions of lives. However, there are so many ways to heal our bodies naturally, and with fewer side effects than pharmaceuticals. Since the beginning of humankind, cultures around the world have utilized herbal remedies for the various therapeutic purposes.

Now known as Phytotherapy, medicinal plants are used to heal and restore balance and wellness within the body - an ancient art that is slowly gaining more respect and interest in the West.

CHAPTER 7: HERBAL REMEDIES FOR BETTER HEALTH AND HORMONE BALANCE

Some plants have truly amazing healing properties and certain botanical extracts and blends can help increase energy, improve your mood, reduce anxiety, help you sleep better, and naturally balance hormones to name a few benefits.

Many conventional prescription drugs available today have roots in the plant world, however, pharmaceutical companies may change the chemical structure of the compound to patent the medications and sell as their unique product and at a much higher price. That is why many herbal remedies and all-natural products are generally not supported my most of the medical industry.

There is a great deal of money in manufacturing, distributing and prescribing pharmaceuticals - even if they have a long list of possible side effects.

Many processed foods and other consumables, as well as over the counter medicines and synthetic topical products contain harmful preservatives, parabens, glycol and other petrochemicals that have been linked to causing cancer and numerous other serious health issues.

By avoiding these types of products and choose a more healthy organic diet with raw fresh ingredients and using all natural products as much as possible, you will be much healthier and have a stronger immune system to fight off disease.

Here are some recommended beneficial botanical extracts that can help support healthy aging and a holistic approach for women to feel better physically, mentally and emotionally.

Sometimes taking a special blend of specific herbs is more effective than each individually. It is also important to know how to properly extract the therapeutic qualities and how much to take.

1. Fenugreek Seed supports healthy hormone levels, improves body composition (increased lean body mass, enhanced muscles, diminished visceral fat), and improves mood and mental cognition.

2. Cordyceps is an extremely effective and powerful life-enhancing mushroom extract used by millions of people worldwide to improve their energy and vitality level and to promote respiratory, circulatory, sexual and immune health.

3. Maitake benefits immune and cardiovascular health.

4. Damiana is effective in relieving anxiety and stress.

5. American Ginseng enhances immune functions and is used by athletes for overall body strengthening. It also strengthens the adrenal and reproductive glands.

6. Maca is growing in world popularity due to its energizing effects and fertility enhancement qualities. Other traditional uses include increasing energy, stamina, and endurance in athletes, promoting mental clarity, and reducing chronic fatigue syndrome.

7. Wulinshine has been proven to alleviate insomnia and depression.

8. Passionflower helps keep your body and mind balanced and reduces anxiety.

9. Black Cohosh has long been known to Native Americans and is used to relieve menstrual cramps and reduce hot flashes.

10. Chasteberry has been used widely in Europe for gynecologic conditions such as premenstrual syndrome (PMS), cyclical breast discomfort, and menstrual cycle irregularities.

11. Red Clover has been used in the treatment of a number of conditions associated with menopause, including hot flashes, cardiovascular health, and osteoporosis.

12. Black Cohosh, Chasteberry, and Red Clover are all called "phytoestrogen" because they're structurally similar to estrogen. Modern scientific studies have shown that these natural herbs contain isoflavones ~ plant-based chemicals that produce estrogen-like effects in the body.

13. Dong Quai helps relieve constipation, increase red blood cell count (which helps treat anemia), and provides relief from menstrual disorders such as cramps, irregular menstrual cycles, infrequent periods, premenstrual syndrome (PMS), and menopausal symptoms.

CHAPTER 8:

HERBAL MEDICINE IS PEOPLE'S MEDICINE

Herbal medicine is people's medicine. Herbal medicine is the primary medicine of most people on this planet, right now. It's not something old and dusty.

It's not a bunch of doctors and chemists figuring out how to use herbs like drugs. Herbal medicine is a 3-year-old picking plantain and putting it on a skinned knee or an insect bite. Herbal medicine is the medicine of women and children. It is the medicine of the earth.

It's medicine that's free. It's not something that must be studied before it can help you. Start with one plant. Approach herbal medicine directly, hands on, in the back yard with your children.

You can be your own herbalist if you keep it simple. First, divide herbs into four categories: nourishing, detoxifying, stimulating/sedating, and potentially poisonous.

Use nourishing herbs daily, unifying herbs regularly, stimulating/sedating rarely, and potentially poisonous herbs almost never.

1. Nourishing herbs are nutritive plants such as kale, garlic, dandelion greens, rolled oats, plantain seeds, blueberries, and edible weeds - the powerhouses of nutrition. Nourishing plants can be used in any quantity for any length of time.

2. Nutritive herbs are rich in minerals and vitamins. One hundred grams of dandelion (about ½ cup of greens) have 14,000 IU of vitamin A.

3. Tonifying herbs are like exercise; they include such plants as burdock, dandelion root, yellow dock, motherwort, ginseng, astragalus, chaste berry, schizandra. One of the benefits of exercise, of tonification, is that it helps us when we're stressed.

You're not necessarily going to feel better if you exercise once for ten minutes. But, if you exercise for ten minutes every day, after several months, you will notice changes.

What's confusing is the difference between tonifying and stimulating herbs. When we take tonics, we feel better and have more energy. When we take stimulating herbs, we also feel better and have more energy, but only when we are stimulating ourselves.

There are immediately uncomfortable effects when we lack our stimulant, but no decrease in health if we stop taking the tonic. Ginger and cinnamon certainly have their uses. But they don't build health.

Over the long run, stimulants erode our health. Nourishing ultimately gives us more energy, though it will take a few days to feel it, whereas the effects of stimulants are immediate.

With nourishing and detoxifying herbs in our daily lives, we have solid energy that adds to health instead of subtracting from it. Instead of raiding my storehouse with stimulants, I build my reserves with nourishing herbal infusions.

I recommend that people drink nourishing herbal infusions on a daily basis. Everything will follow from there.

I consider dark chocolate an important health food.

Stimulating/sedating herbs are some of the most widely used of all herbs? They include coffee, tea, cinnamon, ginger, hops, kava, licorice, passionflower, skullcap, valerian, willow, and wintergreen. They are best used when there is a specific need: A pre-diabetic might choose to take a teaspoonful of cinnamon daily. Ginger compresses are great, and I enjoy it in my food, occasionally. The point with these herbs is to avoid daily use.

The last category is potentially poisonous herbs, ones we only in extreme situations, to ward off death. I include goldenseal, poke root, cayenne, rue, sweet clover, and wormwood in this category.

Goldenseal is a broad spectrum antibacterial. It kills more gut flora than antibiotics. It negatively impacts kidney, liver, and gut function.

When you read about herbal medicine, for instance, or see a doctor or healer, you could ask yourself; The Scientific Tradition says herbs are dangerous; they are crude drugs, drugs with green coats. Drugs have been made from herbs, but that doesn't mean all herbs are drug-like. The Heroic Tradition says herbs - like cayenne, Goldenseal, and Lobelia - cleanse.

We do not fall from that perfection, but we fall from our belief in that perfection. The Heroic Tradition encourages us to berate ourselves, to believe that any health problem is our own fault.

There is power in those beliefs, but little healing, to my mind. To me, healing is healing.

To heal is to make someone more, not less. I strive not to take away, but to add, and let what isn't needed to go as it will, and it will.

We recognize our wholeness/health/holiness when we accept ourselves exactly as we are, with love and compassion. We nourish what we want to be, rather than rejecting what we don't want. We trust our bodies, we trust the earth, and we trust our gut feelings.

Cholesterol's connection to heart attacks has never been proven. And we have virtually no idea what healthy cholesterol is in a post-menopausal woman. Someone may incredibly have high cholesterol, but never had a heart attack.

Inflammation has been shown, over and over, to lead to heart attacks. You may want to consider reducing inflammation instead of cholesterol. One of the best ways to do that is to stop eating oils pressed from seeds, and to start eating olive oil, organic butter, and the natural fats from organically raised, pastured animals.

Canola oil, flax oil, hemp oil, evening primrose oil, soy oil, sesame oil, almond oil, corn oil - all considered healthy, but examples of the oils you avoid when you want to avoid inflammation.

And inflammation underlies and supports heart attack, joint pain, dementia, cancer.

The Scientific Tradition says "measure and fix." For optimal health follow an anti-inflammatory diet - the first step is to remove seed oils from your diet. Then, reduce and remove stimulants - coffee, black pepper, cayenne, ginger, cinnamon, soda pop.

Third, reduce and remove all sources of high-fructose corn syrup. Meanwhile, introduce optimally nutritive foods: nourishing herbal infusions, plain yogurt, fermented vegetables, whole grains, miso, and seaweed. Give yourself at least a year to make these changes. You are already perfect, and you can create a greater perfection as you nourish yourself.

Slippery elm, is a wonderful herbal ally. You make lozenges by mixing slippery elm bark powder with a little honey.

You stir until it clumps up, adding more honey if needed. It's just right when it's like pie dough. Using your hands, you make balls the size of hazelnut or bigger, and roll them in more powdered slippery elm so they don't stick to each other.

You store them in a small metal tin, and don't leave home without it. Slippery elm, is so safe that you can dissolve a ball in your mouth as often as you want, any time you feel any distress.

If you're working with an ongoing condition, at least two a day is good. Slippery elm restores the lining of the intestines, prevents any agents within the body from disturbing the intestines, and neutralizes any poisons that are present in or around the intestines.

A great ally that you could grow is comfrey. There is some controversy about the use of comfrey root, so I restrict myself to the leaf. Also, I'm careful to use garden comfrey, which is less problematic.

To make a nourishing herbal infusion with comfrey, weigh out one ounce of dried leaves and put that in a quart canning jar. Fill it to the top with boiling water.

Screw a tight lid on it and let it steep for at least 4 hours - or up to 9 hours at cool room temperature. Strain the herb out, squeezing it well. The liquid is what we drink; you put the spent herb in the compost. Comfrey leaf infusion can be drunk hot, with a spoonful of honey, or over ice. You can also heat it up and pour it over a mint tea bag. Comfrey gives the lining of the lungs and the intestines flexible strength and health.

Comfrey leaf infusion is good for people who have quit smoking, or even if they are still smoking. Comfrey leaf infusion is also a tremendous ally to bone flexibility and strength.

It also heals and strengthens tendons and ligaments. Remember comfrey: it contains proteins that create short-term memory cells.

Teas and infusions are generally safe; tinctures are more concentrated and thus less safe, and capsules are the least safe of all. In fact, herbs in capsules are the most likely to create horrible side-effects.

Let's go back to our four categories - nourishing herbs contain vitamins and minerals, proteins and nutritive factors that are easily soluble in water and vinegar, but not alcohol.

Stimulating/sedating and potentially poisonous herbs contain active ingredients that are more soluble in alcohol than in water. Thus, infusions and vinegar are nutritive, while tinctures are more drug-like.

An infusion is a large amount of dried herb brewed for a long time. A tea is a small amount of fresh or dried herb brewed for a short time. To make an infusion:

Buy dried herbs in bulk - my favorites for nourishing infusions are stinging nettle, oat straw, red clover, linden, and comfrey leaf - and place one ounce of dried herb in a quart canning jar; fill with boiling water; screw on a tight lid; steep for at least 4 hours; strain; drink the liquid hot or cold; refrigerate what's left and consume it within 36 hours.

A quart of nettle infusion can have 2000mg of calcium, and we could easily consume that in a day. A dropper full of nettle tincture would contain, at the most, 3-5mg of calcium.

The definition of a tincture is an alcohol extract. The active principles in plants - alkaloids, glycosides, volatile oils, and resins - generally dissolve poorly in water. Tinctures can make a plant act more like a drug, and allow finer control over the dose.

Legal Disclaimer: This content is not intended to replace conventional medical treatment. Any suggestions made and all herbs listed are not intended to diagnose, treat, cure or prevent any disease, condition or symptom.

Personal directions and use should be provided by a clinical herbalist or another qualified healthcare practitioner with a specific formula for you. All information in this book is provided for general information purposes only and should not be considered medical advice or consultation.

Contact a reputable healthcare practitioner if you are in need of medical care. Exercise self-empowerment by seeking a second opinion.

CHAPTER 9

HERBAL TEA; HERBAL TEA AND ITS BENEFITS

World of herbal teas extends beyond our imaginations. Teas have been common taste worldwide. Since time immemorial herbal teas are the part of humanity and have been an accompanying him in all his occasions and emotions.

This herbal tea has the origin in the eastern part of the world, i.e. Japan, China, and India. Though initially it was given by herbalist as a medication for treating various ailments, but slowly and gradually it developed the tastes.

Hence, these herbal teas serve two purposes. Firstly, it serves as a medication and supports the health of our body.

Secondly, it acts a natural drink and is pleasing to our tastes. There is countless herbal tea available in the markets. These are created seeking different tastes and requirements of the individual for individuals.

We are proud to present to you our complete range of herbal teas that has been conceptualized on the ideology of Ayurveda and Chinese medicines. These are also prepared by keeping in mind the tea lovers.

CHAPTER 9 HERBAL TEA; HERBAL TEA AND ITS BENEFITS

We have all the basic brands of teas that are made for your requirements. We have

1. Arjun herbal tea: Arjun or Arjuna tea is an herbal tea that will nourish our heart and make us cure of all kinds of heart-related problems. Arjun tea has a component of Arjuna that has now been a world renowned herb for treating all kinds of heart abnormalities. It contains no added sugar and is completely safe for diabetic patients.

2. Digest herbal tea: Digest tea is an herbal tea that will maintain your digestion to the optimized levels. It is based on the Ayurvedic formulation and will help you in reviving your old digestive powers so that you are able to extract maximum energies from the food you eat.

    It will also solve your problems of indigestion, flatulence, and constipation.

3. Green herbal tea: Green tea is an herbal tea that will rejuvenate you and will make you relieved from all your tiredness and fatigue. Green tea will make you relax and would relieve from all the problems you are facing. Its unique anti-aging formulation will always keep you young and will put into you the powers of youth.

4. Kof herbal tea: Kof tea is an herbal tea that has been creating to make you relieved from all your respiratory tract problems. Kof tea will not only help you to recover from all the cough and cold problems, but will also tone up your throat and make your immunity strong to face any infections.

5. Laxa herbal tea: Laxa tea is an herbal tea that has been specially designed to cope up your constipation problem. Laxa tea will ease the peristaltic movements and facilitates the easy evacuation of the bowel.

6. Lean herbal tea: An herbal tea that has been creating waves in the world due to its excellent results in making you lose weight. An Ayurvedic formulation of the herbal tea helps you in easy weight loss in a short span of time.

7. Stress herbal tea: Stress herbal tea is a unique formulation that is very helpful in relieving you from your stressful condition. Stress tea helps in opening up of all the body channels and then evacuates harmful stress builder chemicals that are the main cause of stress.

8. Sleep herbal tea: An Ayurvedic herbal tea that is one of the best and the safest way to induce sleep. It's a natural product which is not a habit forming. It's completely safe for your health.

BENEFITS OF HERBAL TEA AND HERBAL PRODUCTS

Herbal tea, unlike regular tea, is a blend of herbs rather than tea bush leaves. It is made from fresh or dry leaves, roots, seeds, fruits and flowers of therapeutic herbs.

There is huge a variety of herbal teas such as - Catnip, Licorice, Hibiscus, Thyme, Nettle, Rose hip, Chamomile, Yarrow, Fennel, Mint and much more.

Like other herbal products, herbal tea is good for health. It has soothing properties and can also act as an energy drink.

The herbal teas offer diverse health benefits, such as strengthening the nervous system, averting cough and cold, promoting sleep, boosting the immune system, aiding digestion, protecting body cells from damage and warding off depression.

HOW TO BUY HERBAL PRODUCTS

1. Buying herbal products online

If you are looking to buy herbal products online, you have to shop around carefully and pay close attention to the quality, ingredients, manufacturers and date of expiration.

There are definitely good quality products available on the Internet but the opposite is true as well. Do your research. The more extensive research you do, the better a product you are going to find.

2. Finding trustworthy herbal manufacturers

A good way to find reliable herbal manufacturers is to ask the people you know. Talk to your friends and family and learn about some of the most reputed herbal manufacturers. Ask them whether they have personally used herbal products of those manufacturers.

3. Paying attention to the composition

Pay attention to the composition of the product to know if the quantities of ingredients are good for you. Some herbal manufacturers mix harmful base ingredients or excipients in their herbal products; make sure yours is devoid of such ingredients. If you do not know about an ingredient, find out whether it is good or harmful for your health.

4. Sticking to the recommended dosage

Similar to traditional medicine, herbal products should always be taken in the prescribed quantities. Whether you are buying herbal tea or herbal supplements or other herbal items, always adhere to the recommended dosage.

5. Checking the location where the product was made

You must check the herbal manufacturer's factory address because manufacturing standards and quality standards are different in every country. Checking the location where the product was manufactured and shipped from gives you an idea about its quality and reliability.

6. Consulting an expert

Before taking herbal products or herbal tea, it is important to talk to an expert. The person doesn't have to be a professional, but he/she has to have relevant knowledgeable about the same.

The expert would advise you on whether it is alright for you to take herbal supplements if you are already on some regular medication.

CHAPTER 10:

BE YOUR OWN HERBAL EXPERT

Herbal medicine is the medicine of the people. It is simple, safe, effective, and free. Our ancestors used - and our neighbors around the world still use - plant medicines for healing and health maintenance.

It's easy. You can do it too, and you don't need a degree or any special training. Ancient memories arise in you when you begin to use herbal medicine.

This chapter is designed to nourish and activate those memories and your inner herbalist so you can be your own herbal expert.

BE YOUR OWN HERBAL EXPERT USING

1. HONEY

Honey has been regarded as a healing substance for thousands of years. Greek healers relied on honey water, vinegar, water, and honey/vinegar water as their primary cures. An Egyptian medical text dated to about 2600 BCE mentions honey 500 times in 900 remedies.

What makes honey so special? First, honey is antibacterial. It counters infections on the skin, in the intestines, in the respiratory system, or throughout the body.

Second, honey is hydroscopic, a long word meaning "water loving". Honey holds moisture in the place where it is put; it can even draw moisture out of the air. A honey facial leaves skin smooth and deliciously moist.

These two qualities - anti-infective and hydroscopic - make honey an ideal healer of wounds of all kinds, including burns, bruises and decubita (skin ulcers), an amazing soother for sore throats, a powerful ally against bacterial diarrhea, and a counter to asthma.

Third, honey may be as high as 35 percent protein. This, along with the readily available carbohydrate (sugar) content, provides a substantial surge of energy and a counter to depression.

Some sources claim that honey is equal, or superior, to ginseng in restoring vitality.

Honey's proteins also promote healing, both internally and externally. And honey is a source of vitamins B, C, D and E, as well as some minerals. It appears to strengthen the immune system and help prevent (some authors claim to cure) cancer.

Honey is gathered from flowers, and individual honey from specific flowers may be more beneficial than a blended honey. Tupelo honey, from Tupelo tree blossoms, is high in levulose, which slows the digestion of the honey making it more appropriate for diabetics.

Manuka honey, from New Zealand, is certified as antibacterial. My "house brand" is a rich, black, locally-produced autumn honey gathered by the bees from goldenrod, buckwheat, chicory, and other wildflowers.

Raw honey also contains pollen and propolis, bee and flower products that have special healing powers.

Bee pollen, like honey, is a concentrated source of protein and vitamins; unlike honey, it is a good source of minerals, hormonal precursors, and fatty acids. Bee pollen has a reputation for relieving, and with consistent use, curing allergies and asthma.

The pollens that cause allergic reactions are from plants that are wind-pollinated, not bee-pollinated, so any bee pollen, or any honey containing pollen, ought to be helpful. One researcher found an 84 percent reduction in symptoms among allergy sufferers who consumed a spoonful of honey a day during the spring, summer, and fall plus three times a week in the winter.

Propolis is made by the bees from resinous tree saps and is a powerful antimicrobial substance. Propolis can be tinctured in pure grain alcohol (resins do not dissolve well in 100 proof vodka, my first choice for tinctures) and used to counter infections such as bronchitis, sinusitis, colds, flu, gum disease, and tooth decay.

Note: All honey, but especially raw honey contains the spores of botulinus. While this is not a problem for adults, children under the age of one year may not have enough stomach acid to prevent these spores from developing into botulism, a deadly poison.

HERBAL HONEYS

Herbal honey is made by pouring honey over fresh herbs and allowing them to merge over a period of several days to several months. When herbs are infused into honey, the water-loving honey absorbs all the water-soluble components of the herb, and all the volatile oils too, most of which are anti-infective. Herbal honey is medicinal and they taste great. When I look at my shelf of herbal honey, I feel like the richest person in the world.

USING YOUR HERBAL HONEY

Place a tablespoonful of your herbal honey (include herb as well as honey) into a mug; add boiling water; stir and drink. Or, eat herbal honey by the spoonful right from the jar to soothe and heal sore, infected throats and tonsils. Smear the honey (no herb, please) onto wounds and burns.

MAKE AN HERBAL HONEY

Coarsely chop the fresh herb of your choice (leave garlic whole).

Put chopped herb into a wide-mouthed jar, filling almost to the top.

Pour honey, into the jar, working it into the herb with a chopstick if needed.

Add a little more honey to fill the jar to the very top.

Cover tightly. Label.

Your herbal honey is ready to use in as little as a day or two, but will be more medicinal if allowed to sit for six weeks.

Herbal honey made from aromatic herbs makes wonderful gifts.

MAKE A RUSSIAN COLD REMEDY

Fill a small jar with unpeeled cloves of garlic.

If desired, add one very small onion, cut into quarters, but not peeled.

Fill the jar with honey.

Label and cover.

This remedy is ready to use the next day. It is taken by the spoonful to ward off both colds and flu. It is sovereign against sore throats, too. And it tastes yummy!

MAKE AN EGYPTIAN WOUND SALVE

"I thought at first this would be dreadful stuff to put on an open wound ... Instead, the bacteria in the fat disappeared and when pathogenic bacteria were added ... they were killed just as fast," commented scientists who tested this formula found in the ancient Smith Papyrus.

Mix one tablespoonful of honey with two tablespoonfuls of organic animal fat.

Put in a small jar and label.

Increase the wound-healing ability of this salve by using an herbally-infused fat.

MAKE A REMEDY TO COUNTER DIARRHEA

Fill one glass with eight ounces of orange juice.

Add a pinch of salt and a teaspoonful of honey.

Fill another glass with eight ounces of distilled water.

Add 1/4 teaspoonful of baking soda.

Drink alternately from both glasses until empty.

FRESH PLANTS THAT TO USE TO MAKE HERBAL HONEY

Anise hyssop (Agastache foeniculum)

Comfrey leaf (Symphytum off.)

Cronewort/mugwort (Artemisia vulgaris)

Fennel seeds (Foeniculum vulgare)

Garlic (Allium sativum)

Ginger root (Zingiber Officinalis)

Horseradish (Armoracia rusticana)

Lavender (Lavendula off.)

Lemon Balm (Melissa off.)

Lemon verbena (Aloysia triphylla)

Marjoram (Origanum majorana)

Oregano (Origanum vulgare)

Osha root (Ligusticum porterii)

Peppermint (Mentha pipperata)

Rose petals (Rosa canina and others)

Rose hips (Rosa)

Rosemary (Rosmarinus off.)

Sage (Salvia off.)

Shiso (Perilla frutescens)

Spearmint (Mentha spicata)

Thyme (Thymus species)

Yarrow blossoms (Achillea millefolium)

HERBAL SYRUPS

Herbal syrups are sweetened condensed herbal infusions. Cough drops are concentrated syrups. Alcohol is frequently added to syrups to help prevent fermentation and stabilize the remedy. Cough drops and lozenges, having less water, keep well without the addition of alcohol.

Bitter herbs, especially when effective in a fairly small dose, are often made into syrups: horehound, yellow dock, and dandelion, chicory, and motherwort spring to mind in this regard.

Herbs that are especially effective in relieving throat infections and breathing problems are also frequently made into syrups, especially when honey is used as the sweetener: coltsfoot flowers (not leaves), comfrey leaves (not roots), horehound, elderberries, mullein, Osha root, pine, sage, and wild cherry bark are favorites for "a cough" syrups.

USING HERBAL SYRUPS

A dose of most herbal syrup is 1-3 teaspoonfuls, taken as needed. Take a spoonful of bitter syrup just before meal for best results. Take cough syrups as often as every hour.

MAKE AN HERBAL SYRUP

To make an herbal syrup you will need the following supplies:

One ounce of dried herb (weight, not volume)

A clean dry quart/liter jar with a tight lid

Boiling water

Measuring cup

A heavy-bottomed medium-sized saucepan

2 cups sugar or 1½ cups honey

A sterilized jar with a small neck and a good lid (a cork stopper is ideal)

A little vodka (optional)

A label and pen

Place the full ounce of dried herb into the quart jar and fill it to the top with boiling water. Cap tightly. After 4-10 hours, decant your infusion, saving the liquid and squeezing the herb to get the last of the goodness out of it.

Measure the amount of liquid you have (usually about 3½ cups). Pour this into the saucepan and bring to a boil. Reduce the heat until the infusion is just barely simmering.

Continue to simmer until the liquid is reduced by half (pour it out of the pan and into the measuring cup now and then to check).

This step can take several hours; the decoction is not spoiled if it is reduced to less than half, but it is ruined if it boils hard or if it burns. Keep a close eye on it.

When you have reduced the infusion to less than two cups, add the sugar or honey (or sweetener of your choice) and bring to a rolling boil. Pour, boiling hot, into your jar. (Sterilize the jar by boiling it in plain water for a few minutes just before filling it.) If desired, add some vodka to preserve the syrup.

Allow the bottle of syrup to come to room temperature. Label it. Store it in the refrigerator or keep it in a cool place.

MAKE HERBAL COUGH DROPS

You must make a syrup with sugar, not honey to make cough drops, but you can use raw sugar or brown sugar instead of white sugar and it will work just as well.

Instead of pouring your boiling hot syrup into a bottle, keep boiling it. Every minute or so, drop a bit into cold water. When it forms a hard ball in the cold water, immediately turn off the fire.

Pour your very thick syrup into a buttered flat dish. Cool, and then cut into small squares.

A dusting of powdered sugar will keep them from sticking. Store airtight in a cool place.

MAKE THROAT-SOOTHING LOZENGES

Put an ounce of marshmallow root powder or slippery elm bark powder in a bowl.

Slowly add honey, stirring constantly, until you have a thick paste

Roll your slippery elm paste into small balls

Roll the balls in more slippery elm powder

Store in a tightly closed tin. These will keep for up to ten years.

PLANTS THAT CAN BE USE TO MAKE HERBAL SYRUPS

Comfrey leaves (Symphytum uplandica)

Chicory roots (Cichorium intybus)

Dandelion flowers or roots (Taraxacum off.)

Elder berries (Sambucus canadensis)

Horehound leaves and stems (Marrubium vulgare)

Motherwort leaves (Leonurus cardiaca) pick before flowering

Plantain leaves or roots (Plantago majus)

Osha root (Ligusticum porterii)

Pine needles or inner bark (Pinus)

Sage (Salvia off.)

Wild cherry bark (Prunus serotina)

Yellow dock roots (Rumex crispus)

CHAPTER 11:

DIETARY SUPPLEMENTS

A dietary supplement is any product that is intended to supplement the diet and that contains at least one of these ingredients: vitamins, minerals, herbs or other botanicals, amino acids, and substances such as enzymes, organ tissues, glandular, metabolites, or a combination of these ingredients.

If you choose to take a dietary supplement, read the supplement label carefully. The label will show how much of a specific vitamin, mineral, botanical, or other is in each dietary supplement.

The Food and Drug Administration (FDA) and its Center for Food Safety and Applied Nutrition developed regulations for manufacturers in order to help consumers make informed choices when choosing dietary supplements.

Manufacturers are responsible for ensuring that their supplements' facts label and ingredient list are accurate, that the dietary ingredients are safe, and that the content matches the amount declared on the label.

HERE IS THE INFORMATION THAT MUST BE ON A DIETARY SUPPLEMENT LABEL:

- A descriptive name of the product stating that it is a supplement.

- The name and address of the manufacturer, packer, or distributor.

- A list of each ingredient contained in the product, listed in the order of predominance by common name or proprietary blend. Ingredients not listed on the facts panel must appear in the other ingredient statement beneath the panel.

- The net contents of the product.

- The manufacturer's suggested serving size. There are no rules that limit a serving size or the amount of a nutrient in any form of dietary supplements.

- Information on nutrients when they are present in significant levels, such as vitamins A and C, calcium, iron, and sodium, and the percentage Daily Value (% DV) where a reference has been established--this is similar to the nutrients listed in the Nutrition Facts panel on food labels. The Daily Value is essentially the same as the DRI (RDA or AI).

- All other dietary ingredients present in the product, including botanicals and amino acids--those for which no Daily Value has been established.

MULTIPLE AND SINGLE NUTRIENT SUPPLEMENTATION

When you choose a general multivitamin and multi-mineral supplement, consider those that offer the full nutrient spectrum, the full range of B-complex vitamins, and antioxidants like beta-carotene and vitamins C and E. A good rule of thumb is to look for daily value percentage ranges from 50 to 150 percent. If a multivitamin has some but not enough of the other vitamins, you can take additional doses of those particular single supplements.

Typically, a multivitamin cannot hold enough calcium. In addition to this basic multivitamin and mineral supplement, you may want to take single supplements to boost your health for specific conditions. To be sure that you will not be taking excessive amounts over what is already in the basic supplement, subtract the amount in the basic supplement from the larger amount listed for that single supplement.

The difference is the amount of the single supplement you need to add. For example, if your basic supplement provides 200 milligrams (mg) of calcium, you would only take 800 mg of single supplement calcium to receive 1,000 mg of calcium daily.

BOTANICALS COMMON IN HIGH-POTENCY SUPPLEMENTS

Common herbal supplements are sometimes found in the formulation of high-potency or a health-benefit specific multivitamin and mineral supplement. Some herbs are used as specifics and are taken for brief periods or only when symptoms are present.

Some herbs are used as tonics and are taken long term, sometimes with short breaks in between.

For more information on using herbs and their health benefits, read about them from a reliable source and then discuss them with your health practitioner. Become informed!

Here are a few common herbs and their unique properties that you may find in your supplements:

- Ginkgo Biloba (Ginkgo Biloba) is an antioxidant and improves circulation and memory. It may interact with monoamine oxidase (MAO) inhibitors and blood thinners and may cause gastrointestinal upset and headaches.

- Ginseng (Panax ginseng, P. quinquefolius) helps increase energy, and is used as a tonic for fatigue and athletic performance. It may worsen the side effects of stimulants, such as caffeine. Some people experience over-stimulation or stomach upset when taking this herb. Avoid this herb if you have high blood pressure, heart palpitations, insomnia, asthma, or a high fever.

- Siberian Ginseng or Eleuthero (Eleuthero senticosus) helps increase energy and is used as a tonic for fatigue and stress. Its use may increase the effectiveness and side effects of some antibiotics.

- Saw Palmetto (Sernoa repens) is effective in the treatment of prostate enlargement or benign prostatic hyperplasia (BPH). Some people experience stomach upset when taking this herb.

- Echinacea (Echinacea augustifolia, E. pallida, E. Purpurea) is known for its ability to stimulate the body's defenses against minor viral and bacterial infections such as colds and the flu. Persons allergic to the pollen of other members of the aster family, such as ragweed, may also be allergic to Echinacea. Its use may counteract immune-suppressive drugs.

- Green Tea Extract (Camellia Sinensis plant extract) has antioxidant properties, particularly the phytochemical epigallocatechin gallate (EGCG) and is used as a tonic.

- Milk Thistle (Silybum marianum) is considered a liver protector and healer and is used as a liver tonic.

- Black Cohosh (Cimicifuga racemosa) has been shown to be effective for premenstrual and menopausal symptoms, such as hot flashes. It may cause stomach upset. Pregnant and nursing women should avoid using this herb.

CONCLUSION

Natural supplements, on the other hand, are seen more as preventative rather than a cure. Natural remedies can treat both the cause and effect in most cases before they become a serious issue.

As an example, your cholesterol can be managed by using natural supplements, thereby reducing the risk of heart disease or stroke. There are herbal remedies which can address heart health, bone & joint health, digestive health, anti-inflammatory issues, and brain health among others.

The key is to know what you need to do to preempt any major diseases or conditions, many of you do not give heart disease or cancer a second thought unless it affects you directly or someone you love.

How many times you lost someone close to you due to a serious health condition, or watch someone deteriorate from cancer or diabetes and how many times have you watched this occur and say to yourself I don't want that to happen to me? Many of you are sincere about making a lifestyle change after such an event, but don't know how to implement it.

Natural supplements, when administered properly, can give you that change; they can be a benefit to you in ways you cannot imagine.

CONCLUSION

Natural supplements can be used to fortify your body to prevent certain cancers from forming. Natural supplements when properly taken can flush out the toxins in your body which can build up in the liver or digestive system. Natural supplements can be used to strengthen your prostate, lower your cholesterol and keep your blood pressure in check.

All of these conditions can be managed with natural remedies. Today just as with the advances in the pharmaceutical industry, natural supplements or nutraceuticals as some are now called is diligently working to naturally improve upon the age old remedies which had served mankind for centuries.

In fact, this alternative form of treatment is making a comeback because many health care professionals see the benefit of keeping you well rather than treating you when are sick and the best way to accomplish this is the implementation of natural supplements.

So take the next step and consider what you need to do to live longer and healthier.

Finally, if you found this book useful in anyway, a review on Amazon is always appreciated!

Thank you and good luck with your healthy herbs!

www.ingramcontent.com/pod-product-compliance
Lightning Source LLC
Chambersburg PA
CBHW062059280526
45788CB00003B/1286